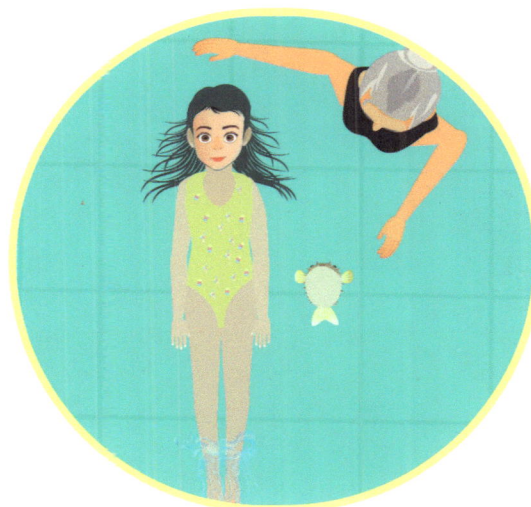

Learn to Swim the Australian Way
Level 2 The Basics
Written by AlyT

Learn To Swim the Australian Way
Level 2 The Basics

Part of the Learn to Swim the Australian Way series with AlyT

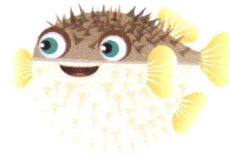

DEDICATED TO

my mother **RHONDA** aka **MRS PAUL**
who taught me everything I needed to know
about life & Jesus †

AND my mentor **PETER TIBBS** aka **TIBBSIE**; both
of whom helped mould me into the swimmer and
swimming teacher I am today.

Formatting: Aluycia Suceng
Editing: Phoenix Raig
Illustrator: PicassoJR
First printing: 2022

Disclaimer
While we draw on our own prior professional expertise and background in the area
of teaching learn to swim, by purchasing and reading our products you acknowledge
that we have produced this book for informational and educational purposes only. You
alone are solely responsible, and take full responsibility for your own wellbeing as well
as the health, lives and wellbeing of your family and children in your care.

www.borntoswim.com.au
SwimMechanics@yahoo.com
Other books by this Author:
Water Awareness Newborns
Water Awareness Babies
Water Awareness Toddlers
Learn to Swim the Australian Way Level 1 – The Foundations

SAFETY FIRST!

* NEVER SWIM ALONE
The non-swimmer should always be accompanied by a responsible adult who can swim.
Where possible, let the lifeguard on duty know you are learning to swim or a beginner swimmer.

* NEVER FORCE A SWIMMER UNDER THE WATER
Learning to swim should be fun & appropriate to the individual's pace.
Whilst not ideal, many activities can be practised with the face out of the water until
the nervous swimmer is ready to submerge their face. Allowing non-swimmers to play
and enjoy the water is crucial to overcoming their fear of the water.

* NEVER HOLD YOUR BREATH FOR EXTENDED PERIODS OF TIME
Hyperventilating and breath holding games are dangerous and can cause you to faint
(lose consciousness) in the water. Search 'shallow water black-out' for more information.

* LEARNING TO SWIM IN SHALLOW, WAIST DEPTH WATER IS BEST FOR BEGINNERS
Until you can confidently move yourself through the water and float comfortably on your back,
beginner swimmers should continue to practise in shallow water only.

A NOTE TO ALL THE SAILORS & SIRENS LEARNING TO SWIM

CONGRATULATIONS on completing the 21 foundational skills from Level 1 – The Foundations!
You've discovered how to enter the water, control your breath, float and balance in various positions, kick with your legs and pull yourself through the water with your arms. Most importantly, you've also learnt **HOW TO BE SAFER** and **MORE CONFIDENT** around water.
Are you ready to have even more fun learning to swim?

Just as in our first book, in Level 2 we'll uncover **21 NEW SKILLS** to help **BUILD MUSCLE MEMORY, IMPROVE BALANCE** and **INCREASE TRACTION & PROPULSION** in the water. You'll start to see the beginnings of the four competitive strokes **(FREESTYLE, BACKSTROKE, BREASTSTROKE AND BUTTERFLY),** and dives & turns start to emerge. We'll also learn some **FUN WATER SAFETY STUFF** along the way too.

For the parents and teachers teaching these skills, ensure your **SWIMMER STUDENT PERFORMS EACH SKILL,** to the best of their ability, **4–5 TIMES EVERY LESSON.** Don't be afraid to correct mistakes and always give **LOTS OF PRAISE AND ENCOURAGEMENT.** For our student swimmers, remember that 'I can't' doesn't exist in the learner swimmer's vocabulary, but **'I'LL TRY' AND A BIT OF EFFORT** always should. Some skills you'll learn in minutes, others may take weeks and months of hard work.
Aim to **POLISH AND REFINE EACH OF THE SWIMMING SKILLS AT EVERY LESSON.** Small adjustments of body position and the use of **VERBAL CUES** will fast track learning and memory recall.

Moving to the next skill before you've properly mastered the current ones, skipping past a skill and the continual practise of a skill with poor form, with no regard to correct body positioning, will lead to bad habits and sloppy swimming. To **ACCELERATE LEARNING,** practise new skills over **SHORT DISTANCES OF 2-3 METERS IN SHALLOW WATER;** practicing newly learnt skills over longer distances leads to fatigue and the new skills and technique will tend to fall apart.

Once again for ease of learning, we've included **VISUAL CUES, CATCHY NAMES** and easy to remember **VERBAL CUES** for each of the skills, and have presented them **IN THE LOGICAL ORDER** we usually perform them during an in-person class. All learner swimmers, teachers and parents should remember to follow the motto to **'LEARN SLOW TO SWIM FAST',** and adhere to the four P's of learning: **PATIENCE, PRAISE, PERFECTION AND PRACTICE.** Yep, I added a new one!

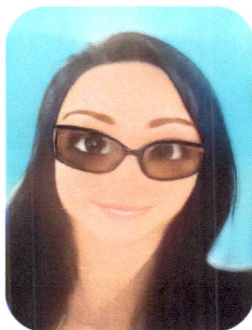

Yours swimmingly,

Alyt

P.S The fastest way to improve your swimming is to **GET IN THE WATER AND PRACTISE OFTEN,** at least 3x a week. See you at the next level!

I CAN DO A STRIDE ENTRY!

A Stride Entry should be used when I don't know the depth of the water or what might be below its surface. When I jump in, I always return to safety or float and wait for help.

I stand on the side of the pool with my toes curled over the edge, my arms out like a pair of aeroplane wings and my hands flat and firm. My eyes are looking at the spot where I want to land, so I don't hit my head or hurt myself on the way in. I lean forward and leap out over the water taking in a big Pufferfish Breath and bend my knees slightly. As I enter the water I use my arms, hands and legs to slow me down and to try and keep the top of my head dry.

I never enter the water **without an adult** who can swim.

1.6 m

Before jumping into the water, I first check:

1 the depth of the water?

2 is there a safe place for me to get in and out of the water?

3 is someone watching and close by to help me if I need them?

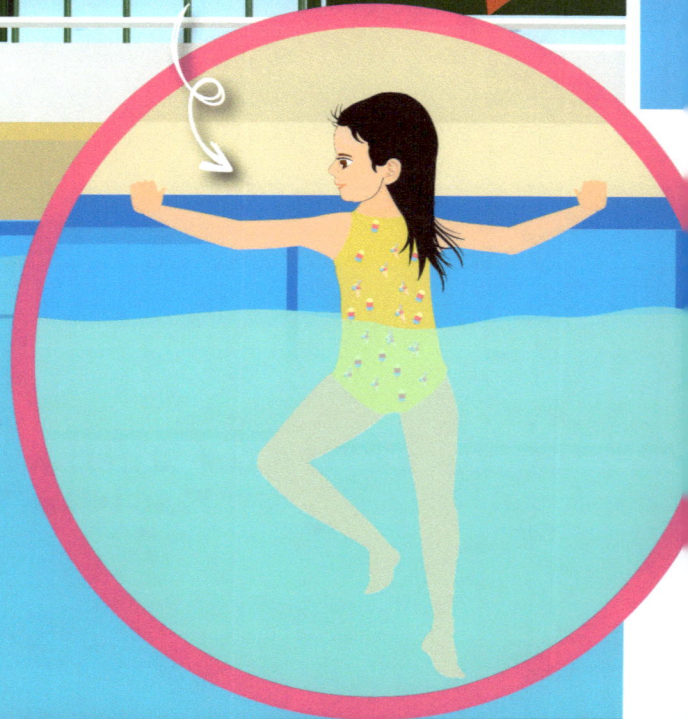

I CAN BLOW BUBBLES!

I hold onto the side of the pool or an adult's hands, take in a big, noisy Pufferfish Breath and seal my lips, trapping the air in my lungs. Then I lower myself into the water and blow the air out of my mouth, like I am blowing out a candle. I try to blow bubbles for the count of 3!

After I blow all the air out under the water, I come up to the surface and take in another quick Pufferfish Breath before going back under and trying again.

Blowing bubbles is a fun way to relax in the water and to exchange old air and new air.

1.2.3!

I CAN BLOW DRAGON BUBBLES!

HUMMM!

Dragon Bubbles are just like regular bubbles except I blow them out of my nose, not my mouth. Blowing bubbles out of my nose when I'm under water stops the water from going up and making me sneeze or feel uncomfortable.

To make Dragon Bubbles, I hold onto the side of the pool or an adult's hand, take a big, noisy Pufferfish Breath and seal my lips. I lower myself into the water and push the air out of my nose like I am blowing into a tissue. It helps if I keep my mouth shut and hum when under the water. I hum for a count of 3!

After I blow all the air out under the water, I come up to the surface, take another noisy, Pufferfish Breath and go back under to try again.

3

I CAN ZOMBIE FLOAT!

Zombie Floats help me to stay relaxed and to balance horizontally in the water. I can practise them with a kickboard until I can float in a perfectly straight line without one.

When I am ready to do them without a kickboard, I start by standing in the water with my arms stretched out in front of me. My hands are floppy with my fingertips tilted downwards slightly, I gently press my thumb against my hand and relax my neck as I look down at the bottom of the pool.

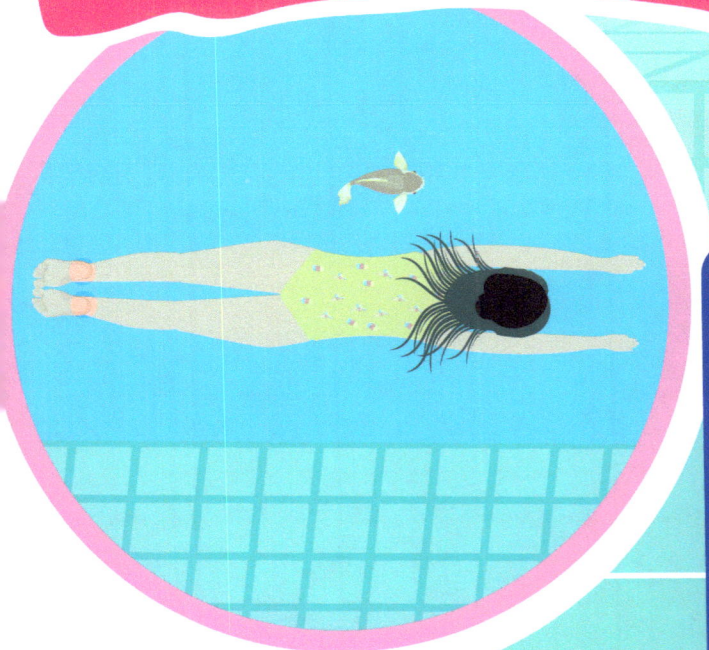

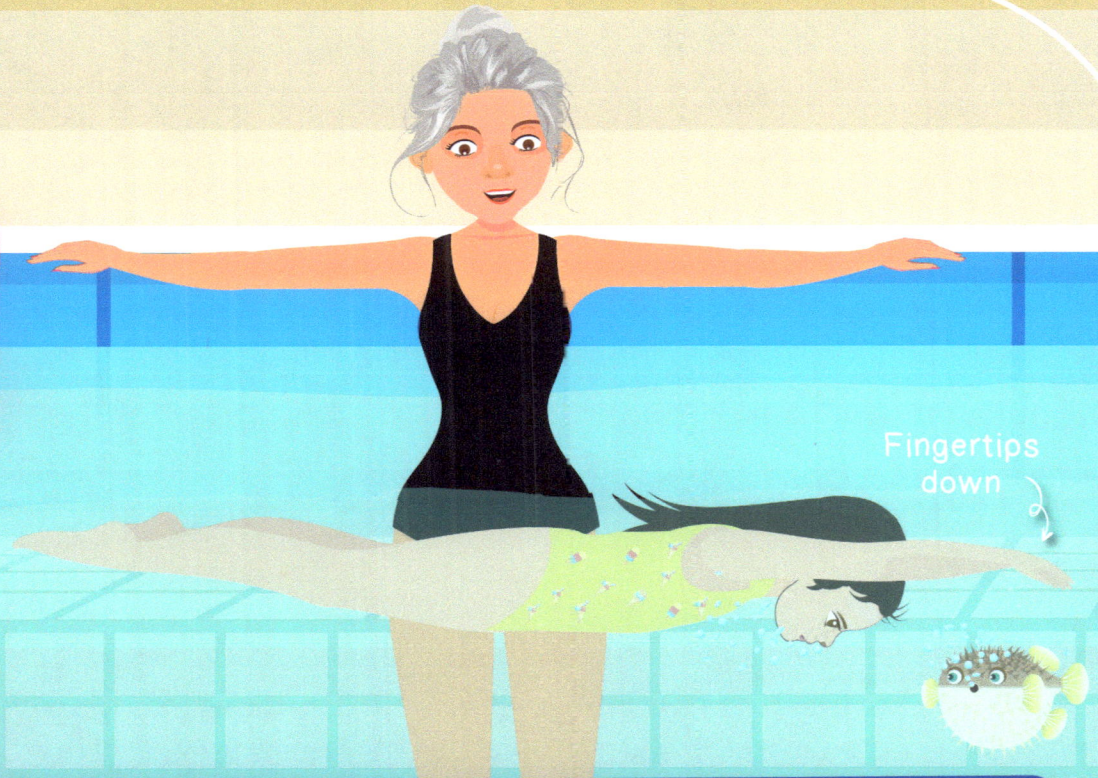

Fingertips down

As I lean forward, I follow my fingertips into the water, I lift one foot off the bottom of the pool and float it up behind me as I gently push off the bottom with the other foot. To float, I keep my eyes looking down and my arms and legs in a straight line with my body. While I float, I focus on staying flat by reaching forward with my arms and stretching my legs out behind me, with only my heels breaking the surface. I angle my feet inwards so my big toes touch and slowly let out bubbles, counting to 10 in my head. Once I have finished, I bend my knees to my chest and sit myself up, planting my feet on the bottom to stand back up.

4

I CAN FLY FLOAT!

The Fly Float is just like a Zombie Float except this time when I stretch my arms out, I turn my hands slightly inwards to angle my thumbs down. My pinky finger stays just under the surface of the water as I float and balance.

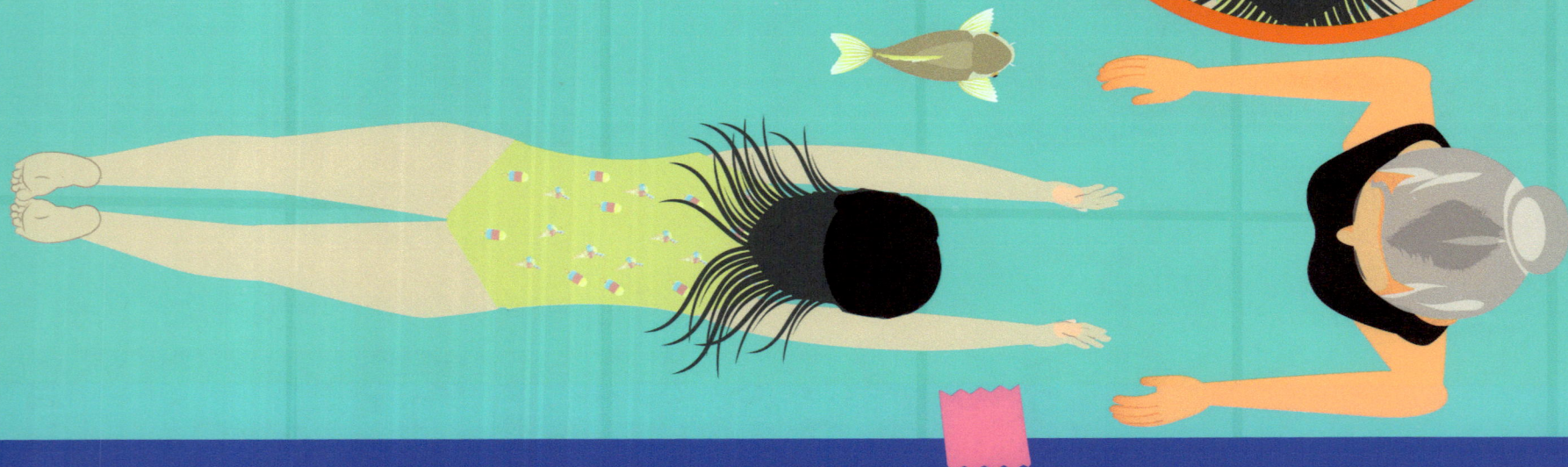

To Fly Float, I lean forward into the water, with my arms stretched out in front of me, and gently push off the bottom of the pool with both feet. I keep my eyes looking down and my arms and legs in a straight line with my body. While I float, I focus on staying flat by reaching forward with my arms, keeping my hands turned inwards with my thumbs down and stretching my legs out behind me with only my heels breaking the surface. I point my toes and angle my feet inwards so my big toes touch and slowly let out bubbles, counting to 10 in my head. To stand back up, I bend my knees and sit myself up, planting my feet firmly on the floor of the pool.

I CAN DEAD FLY FLOAT!

The Dead Fly Float is just like the Zombie Float; except this time my arms are at my sides, not out in front of me.

I stand in the water, lock my arms at my sides with my thumbs pressed against my legs. I lean forward, slowly entering the water face first as I gently push off the bottom of the pool with both feet. I look straight down and float my legs up behind me, keeping them straight and stretched. My heels are out of the water, legs just under the surface and big toes touching as I count in my head to 10!

1..2..3..4..5..6..7..8..9..10!

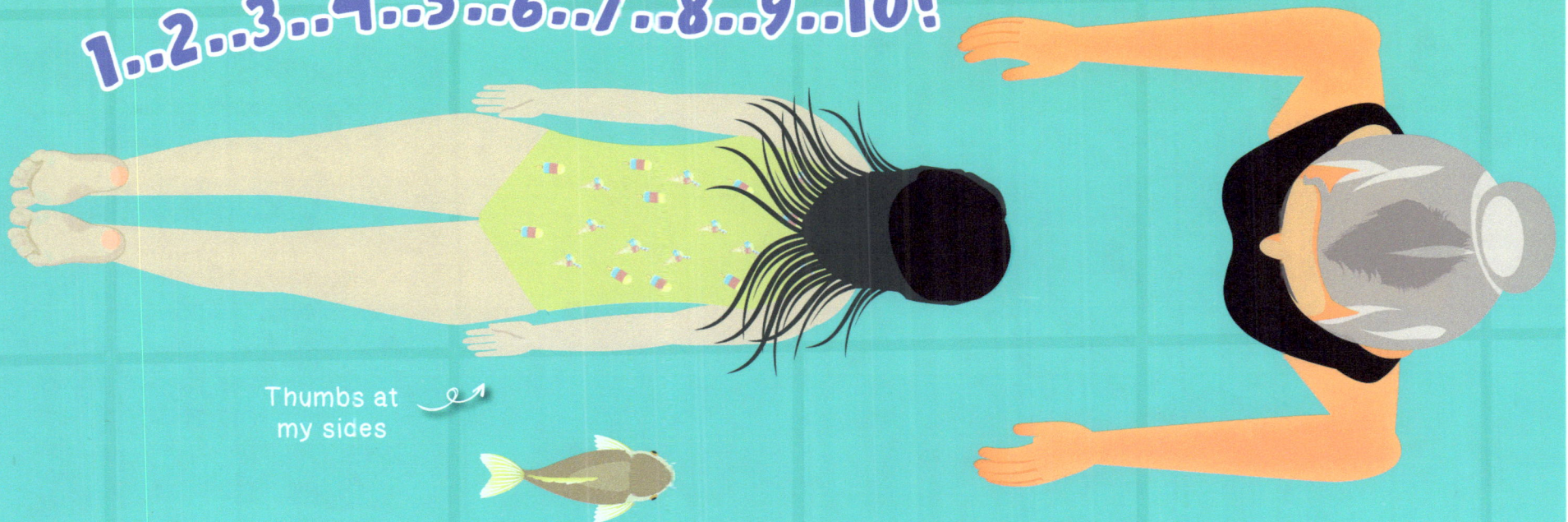

Thumbs at my sides

I CAN FROG FLOAT!

A Frog Float makes my body look like a frog floating in the water, it teaches me to balance in the water with my feet turned out.

I can practise my Frog Float out of the water on the pool deck by laying flat, like a starfish, then bending my knees and lifting my feet up behind me and placing my heels together.

Other ways to practise turning my feet out are by standing up straight and tall and doing a Penguin Pose or sitting on a chair and wrapping my feet around the legs of the chair and stretching my heels down while keeping my knees together.

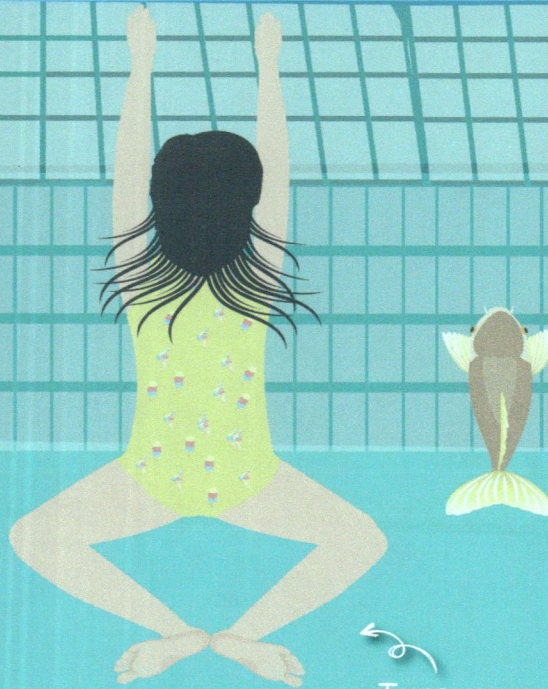

Turn my feet out

To Frog Float in the water, I hold onto the side of the pool or submerged step with my face in the water, looking straight down. Then I Starfish Float my legs up to the surface of the water. Once I am floating, I bend my knees and bring my feet up behind me. I turn my feet outwards and bring my heels together as I relax and count to 3!

I CAN PENCIL FLOAT!

A Pencil Float is a Torpedo Stretch but in the water.

I stand in the water and make a sandwich with my hands, one on top of the other, locking them with my thumbs. Then I stretch my arms up over my head, squeezing the back of my ears with my arms.

I bend my knees and lean forward, slowly entering the water face and fingertips first. As I gently push off the bottom of the pool with both feet pointing behind me, I straighten my legs and float them up behind me. I keep my feet together with my big toes touching.

To ensure I look like a sharp pencil floating at the surface of the water, I keep my arms and hands locked together and stretch out as far as I can without becoming too stiff. If my body becomes too tense, I will start to sink, so I float for the count of ten and blow bubbles to keep myself relaxed.

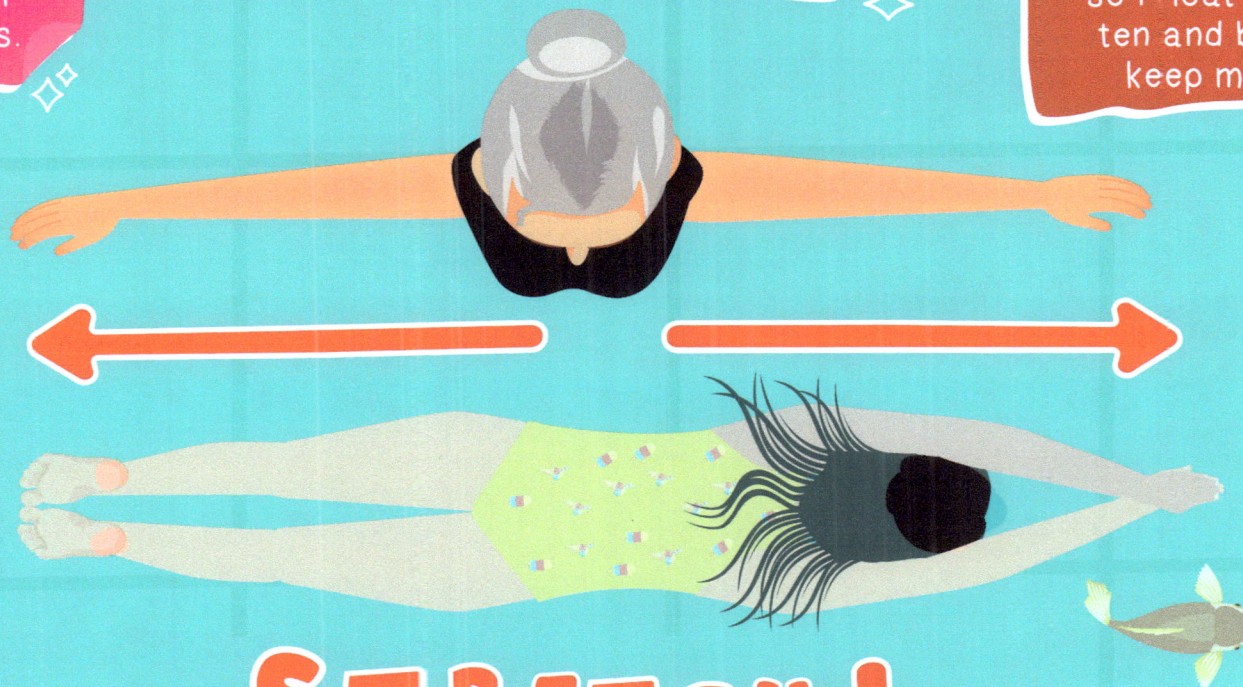

STRETCH!

I CAN BLAST OFF!

Blast Offs help move me through the water quickly by using my legs and feet to push off the sides and bottom of the pool. I also use my Blast Offs from the submerged steps when holding onto a kickboard.

To Blast Off, I Bunny Crouch and balance with my arms and hands locked over my head, like I do when I Torpedo Stretch. I count down from 3-2-1 as I bend my knees and lean forward so I can enter the water hands and face first.

When my countdown reaches 1, I take a Pufferfish Breath in and push off using both my feet and the muscles in my legs. I Blast Off with my eyes looking down, and body in a nice straight line so I can glide across the surface of the water.

As I start to slow down, I separate my hands and push the water behind me by sweeping my arms down past my body to my legs. I blow a long stream of bubbles as I continue to move through the water. When my thumbs touch the sides of my legs I stop and turn around to go back to the other side of the pool where I started.

It is important to remember when doing Blast Offs to not throw myself into the water, otherwise I will jump, flop and sink.

I CAN FLUTTER KICK!

FLOPPY FEET !

I can make my kick stronger by Flutter Kicking my legs when I swim.

I sit on a submerged step and float my legs up to just under the surface of the water. I keep my legs straight, with a small bend in my knees and my toes pointed. I start slow and try to kick the water out of the pool with the top of my feet, making sure my big toes stay close enough to brush past each other as I Flutter Kick.

I keep my feet floppy, not stiff, as I imagine I am kicking my dirty socks off my feet. If my knees pop out of the water, I know I am bending them too much. While I am learning, I can put a kickboard over my knees to remind me to kick with long ballerina kicks, not short bent kicks.

To practise kicking on my belly I lay in shallow water holding onto a submerged step. I let my legs float up behind me, keeping my ankles dry. I press my face in the water and blow bubbles as I count to 6 and do fast little kicks. I kick the water away from me with the soles of my feet and the back of my calves as my big toes stays close to brush past each other. If my knees touch the floor of the pool and my whole foot comes out of the water, I know I am bending my knees too much.

I CAN ROCKET KICK!

Now that I have practised learning how to Flutter Kick, I can add some rocket power to my floats and Blast Offs. My Pencil Float becomes a kick-powered Rocket, shooting across the water.

I begin by Bunny Crouching on a submerged step, locking my hands and squeezing my arms against the back of my ears over my head. I lean forward and enter the water fingertips and face first as I count down and Blast Off.

I look straight down as I keep my hands and arms locked, reaching forward with my fingertips tilted slightly down. I do lots of fast little kicks and my body stays stretched out long until I run out of my rocket-fuel bubbles. After a short rest, I Blast Off and Rocket Kick back to where I started.

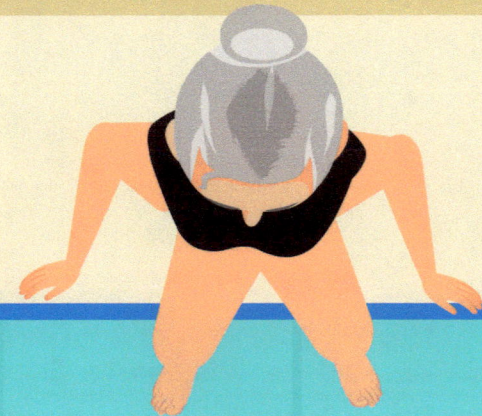

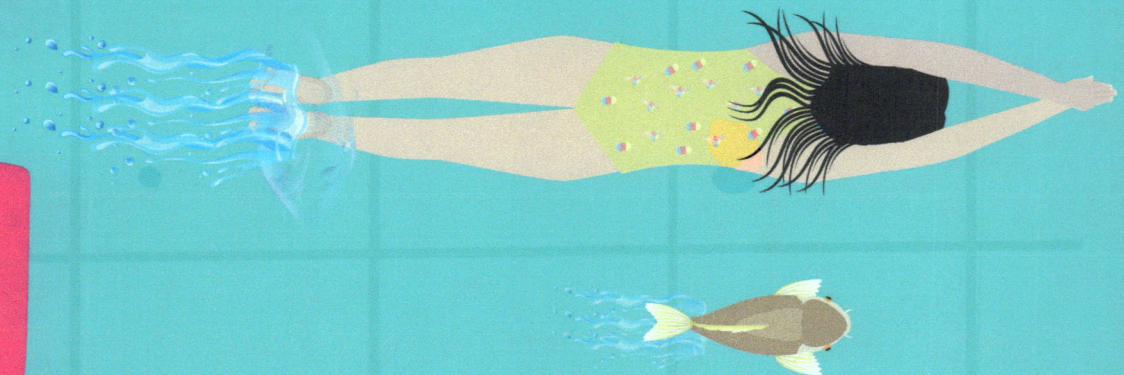

I CAN SOLDIER FLOAT!

Before I do my Soldier Floats in deeper water, I practise them on a shallow ledge. I lay down, like I am laying in bed, and let the water gently lap around me. Sometimes it tickles as the water fills my ears. I lay still and learn to ignore it as I listen to my breathing and the sounds under the water.

To Soldier Float I look straight up at the sky with my arms at my sides and my thumbs touching my legs. I slowly lift my legs off the bottom of the pool by tilting my hips up and using my stomach muscles. My legs float just under the surface of the water, my feet are pointed away from me and my big toes are touching.

When I am ready, I practise in deeper water with an adult helping me. To start my float in the deeper water, I hold onto the side of the pool and tilt my head back until my ears are in the water and I am looking up at the sky. I push off the wall very gently, sweeping my arms in to rest them against my sides. I try to keep my body in the same position I practised in the shallow water, remembering to stay relaxed but not too floppy or too stiff. I use my muscles to adjust my balance so I can float at the surface of the water. I do gentle baby kicks to get back to the wall or back to safety.

Ears Under!

Eyes to the sky!

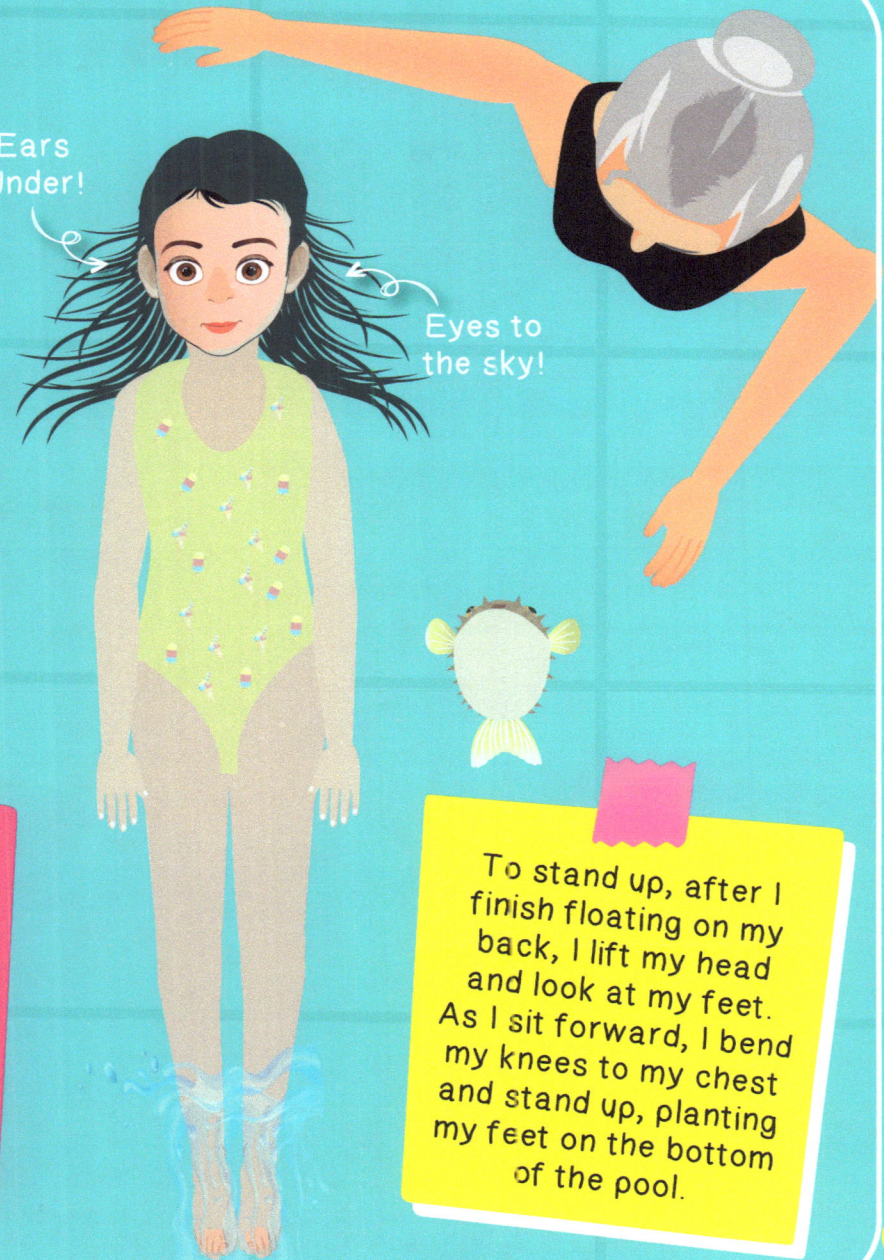

To stand up, after I finish floating on my back, I lift my head and look at my feet. As I sit forward, I bend my knees to my chest and stand up, planting my feet on the bottom of the pool.

I CAN FLIP & KICK!

Now that I know how to float and kick, it's important I learn how to roll over onto my back to get air without having to lift my head which can make my legs sink.

I Blast Off from the side of the pool making sure I am looking straight down and kicking lots of fast little kicks. As I sweep my arms under me, I continue to kick hard and turn my face towards the surface. My arms help me as I roll onto my back, like I am rolling over in bed.

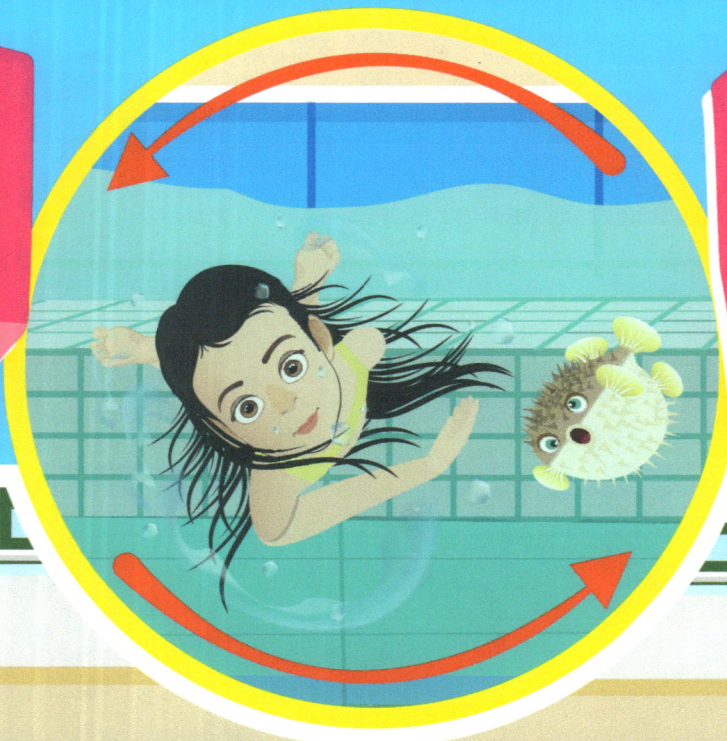

It is important I kick and use my arms to flip me onto my back. As my face breaks the surface, I tilt my head back and look straight up at the sky to get my ears under the water so I can Soldier Float and have a rest. I never look at my feet when I kick or float on my back, otherwise my belly will sink.

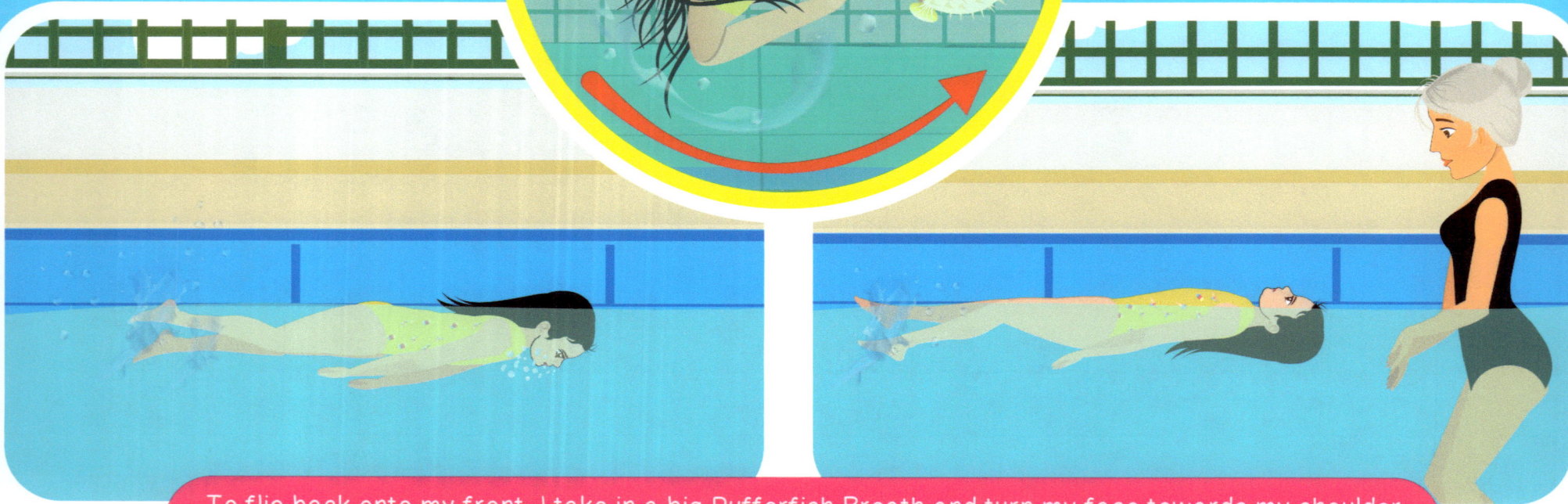

To flip back onto my front, I take in a big Pufferfish Breath and turn my face towards my shoulder and into the water. I continue to Kick & Flip until I reach the pool wall or safety.

I CAN SUPERMAN KICK!

Superman Kicking teaches me to kick in a straight line as I follow my arm out front, called my lead arm. Before adding my kicks, I practise a Superman Float with a kickboard. Holding onto the kickboard and floating helps me to remember to keep my arms in-line with my shoulders.

I stretch my lead arm forward as I Crocodile Hold the kickboard with one hand, keeping a firm grasp. My other arm is at my side with my thumb pressed against my leg. Both my arms stay straight as I add some fast, little kicks.

When I am ready to try without a kickboard, I Blast Off with one arm pressed against my leg and the lead arm straight out in front of me, in-line with my shoulder. I reach forward in the water with my fingertips angled downwards and thumb pressed against my hand. I focus on looking down as I kick and blow bubbles, letting my hand lead me and find the wall.

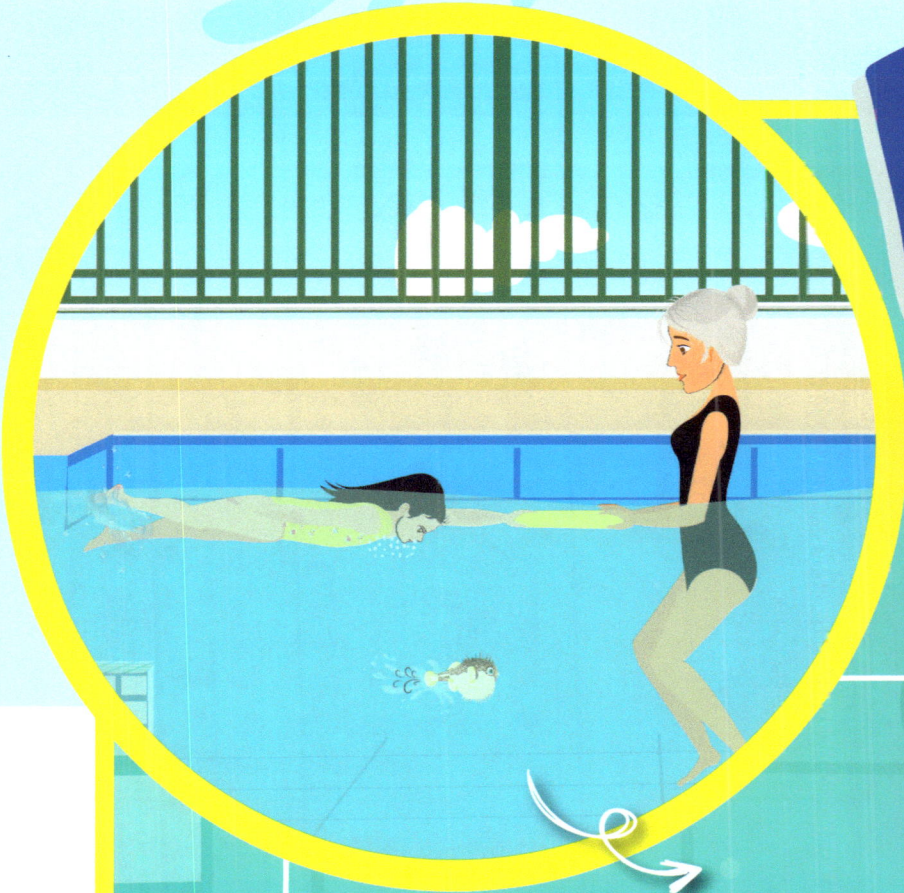

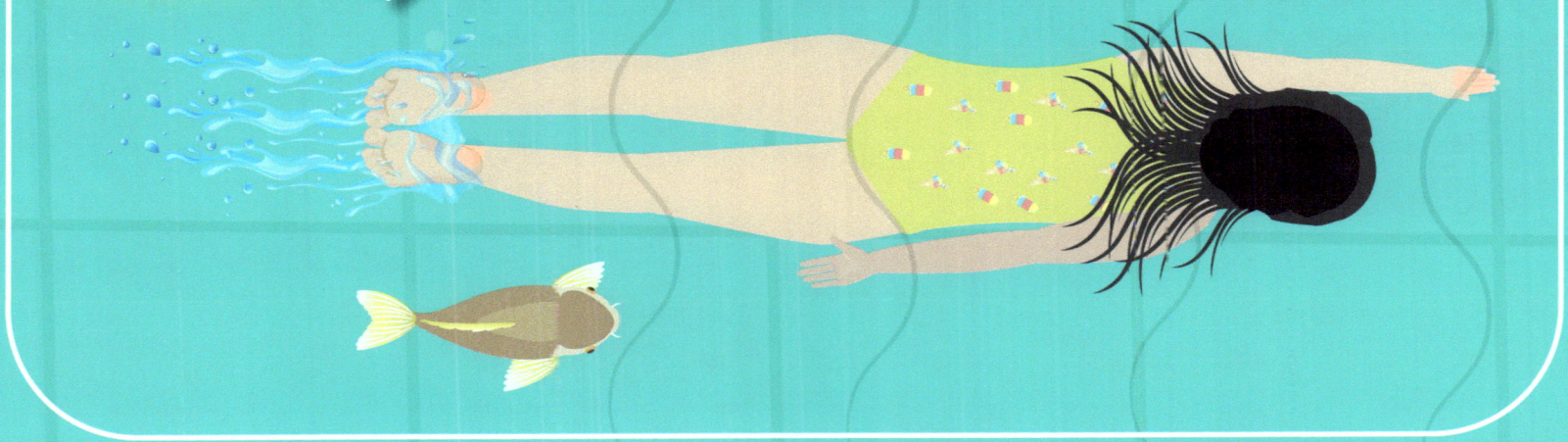

I CAN FREESTYLE MARCH!

I Freestyle March on the pool deck or in shallow water to help remember which direction my arms need to move when I learn Freestyle. It also helps me learn to move my feet and swing my arms at the same time.

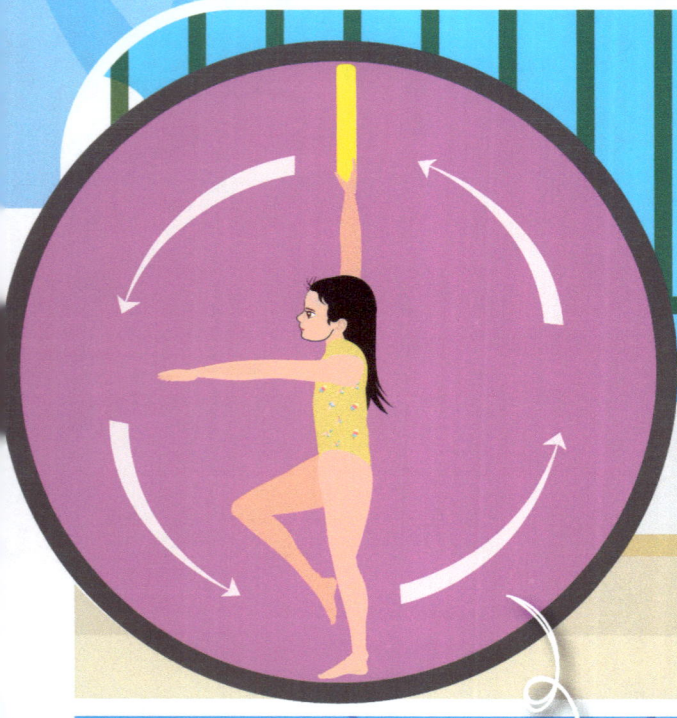

I hold the kickboard with both hands above my head, stretching it up high. My thumb and my fingers firmly hold onto the kickboard in a Crocodile Hold. I let go and sweep one arm straight down to my side. When my thumb touches my leg, I know it is time to swing my arm up and around behind me to grab the kickboard. When my arm touches my ear, I release the kickboard and make another circle using my other arm.

I pretend my arms are the arms of a large clock, taking their turn moving in circles.

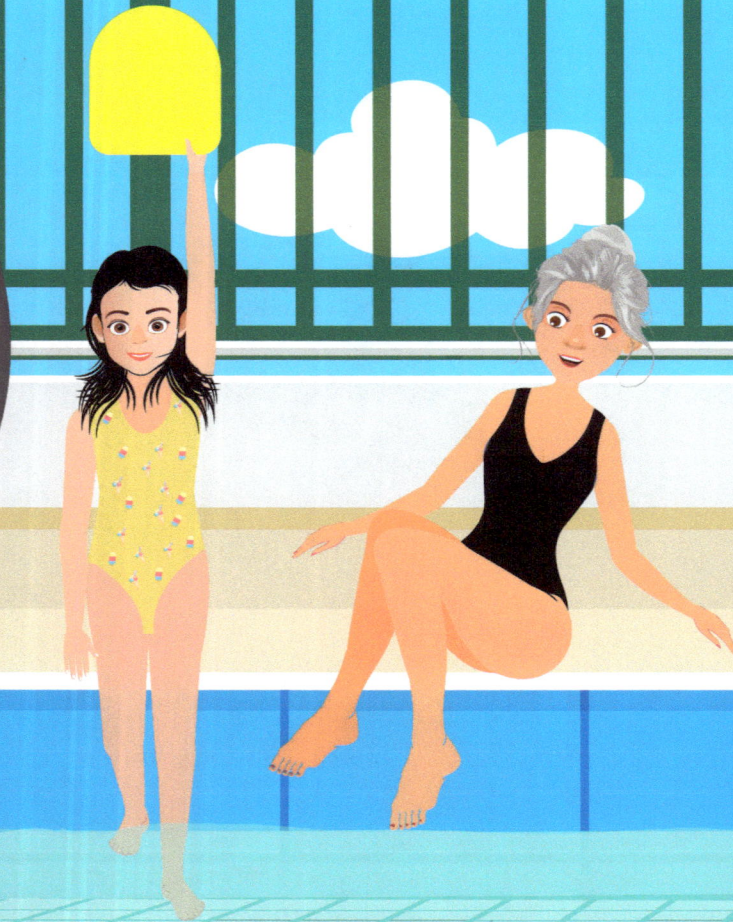

I never look at the kickboard as I Freestyle March, I always keep my eyes looking straight ahead and count four big, slow circle arms.

I CAN DO
SIX KICKS SWITCH!

SWITCH!

123456!

Six Kicks Switch is like the Superman Kick, but this time I kick and swap my lead arm over.

1 I rest my lead arm against my ear as I kick six kicks. To swap my arms I reach my lead arm forwards and sweep it down past my side, pushing the water behind me with my hand, stopping when my thumb touches my leg.

123456!

2 At the same time, my other arm, that is pressed against my side, sweeps over the top of the water. I imagine my arm is a paint brush attached to my armpits. I use a soft, relaxed hand to paint the sky with my fingertips as it goes over. My hand lands in the water fingertips first straight out in front of my shoulder. I do six more kicks and stop so I can have a rest.

SWITCH!

3 I can also practise swapping my arms using a kickboard. It helps if an adult pulls me along so I can concentrate on kicking and switching arms four times, letting both arms take turns holding the kickboard.

123456!

I CAN CATERPILLAR KICK!

For my Caterpillar Kick, I learn to kick with both my feet together at the same time. This kick lets me wriggle through the water like a Caterpillar.

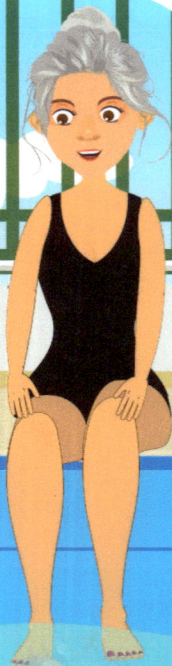

I hold onto the side of the pool or a submerged step and Fly Float, pressing my thumbs downwards to anchor me in place while I float. When I am balanced, I bend my knees slightly and kick both feet downwards pressing the front of my toes against the pressure of the water.

BEND !

FLICK !

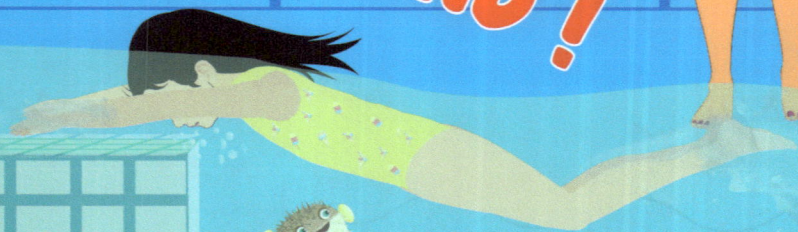

It's important I stay close to the surface of the water when I practise. I do this by keeping my arms straight and looking straight down each time I practise a kick. I also focus on not bending my knees too much, otherwise my hips will drop too deep and I will start to sink making it harder to kick.

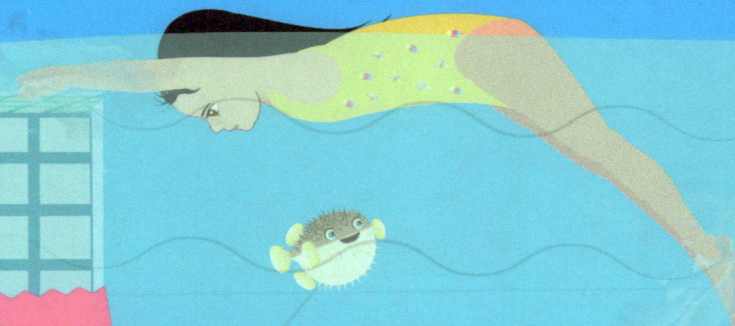

Kicking my feet downwards pushes my bottom up and out of the water. I press my chest down as my legs finish the kick and straighten into an arch, like the tail of a dolphin. I do one kick at a time before stopping to take a breath and restarting each kick until I get it right.

I CAN SEAHORSE BALANCE!

The Seahorse Balance is a fun challenge to help me use my hands and feet in the water to stay upright.

I climb onto a pool noodle, like I am climbing onto a horse and try my best to stay upright by holding onto the side of the pool and the neck of the noodle. As I get better at balancing I hold onto the front of the noodle with both hands. It is important I do not lean too far forward, otherwise I will become unbalanced.

Learning to balance takes practice. I have to use the muscles in my belly and my back. Once I can sit up straight on my seahorse, I challenge myself by turning in a slow circle, using only my feet and legs or only my arms and hands.

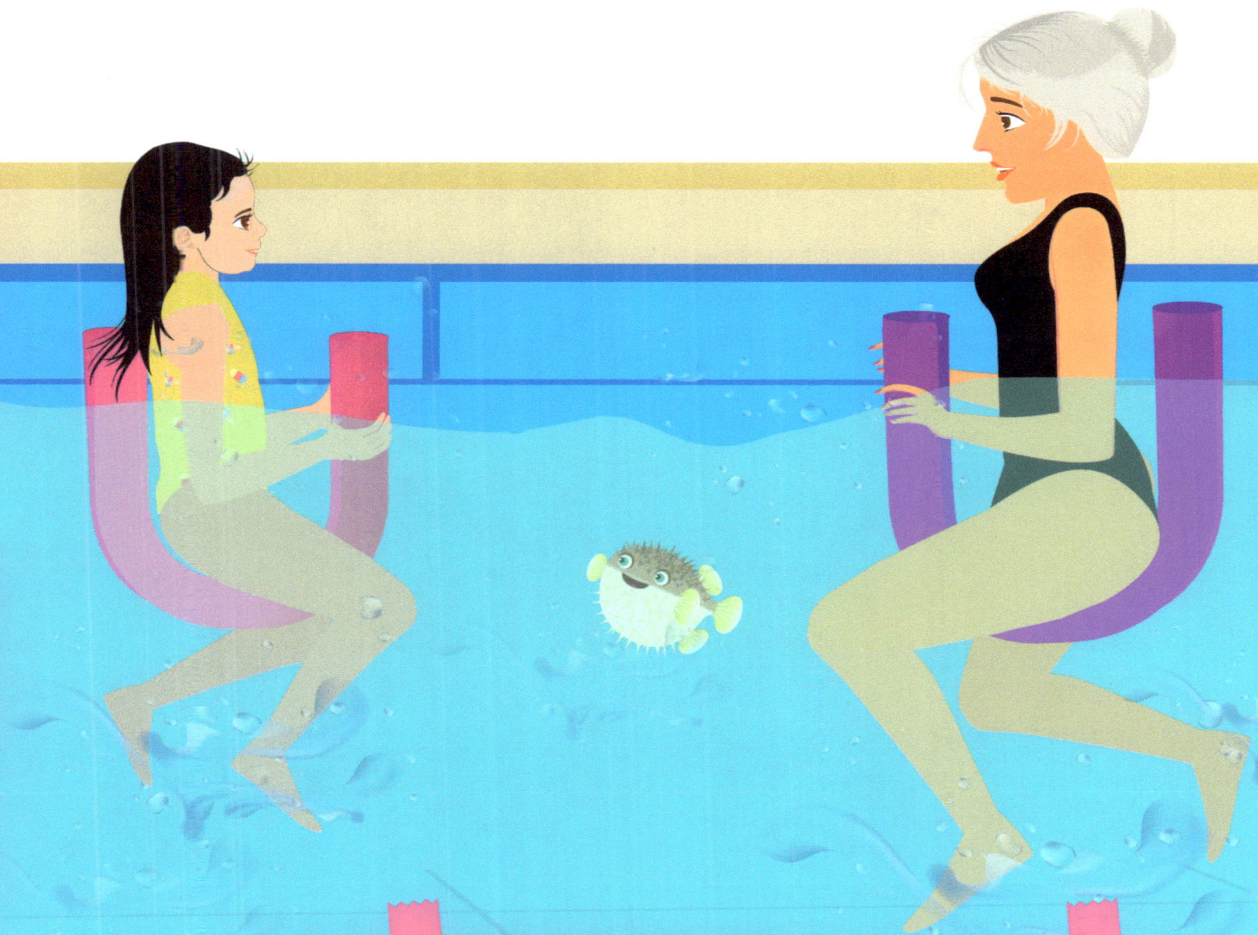

It is important to put pool noodles and other pool toys away when we finish using them. Tripping on toys and reaching for toys in the water can cause others to accidentally fall into the water.

I CAN DO SURVIVAL BACKSTROKE!

I use Survival Backstroke to relax and move quietly across the water on my back. I pretend the fish underneath me are asleep and swim slowly without making a lot of splash so as to not wake them up.

1. I start by Soldier Floating and bending my knees to draw my heels up behind me. Next, I turn my feet out so my legs are Frog Floating, but on my back. As I draw my heels up and together, I zip my thumbs up my sides to my armpits. This is my Chicken Float.

2. From my Chicken Float I spread my arms and legs out into a Starfish Float by turning my knees inwards, straightening my legs and pointing my toes.

3. Once I am Starfish Floating, I quickly snap my legs together, return my arms back to my sides and Soldier Float. I practise each float changing slowly from one to the other.

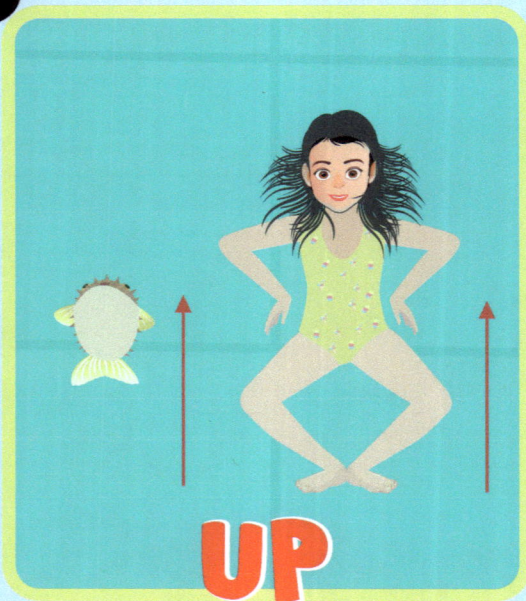

UP

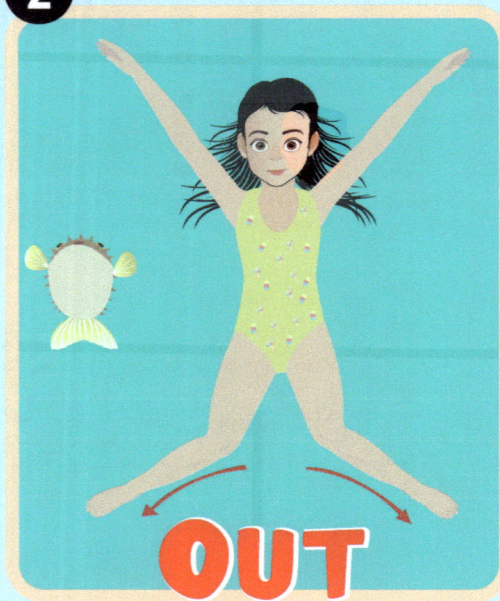

OUT

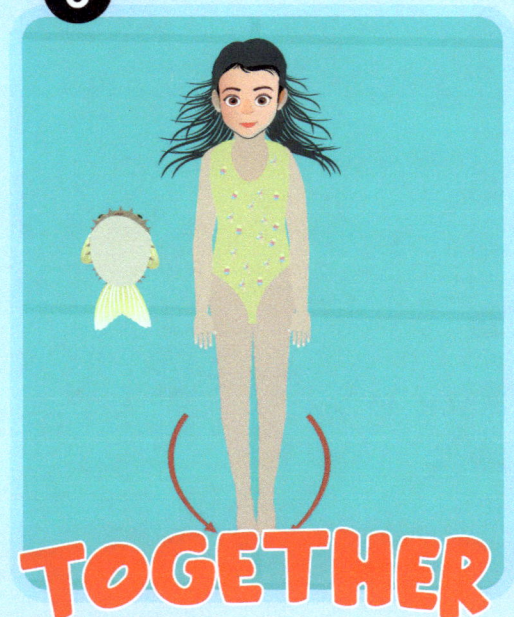

TOGETHER

As I get better at each float, I start to move across the water by pushing the water with my hands and feet and whipping my arms and legs up, out and around. When I snap my legs together my big toes find each other and I pause for a count of 1–2!

I CAN DO A SEATED DIVE!

I sit on the edge of the pool with my knees together and feet pressed against the side. My knees are bent, acting as a wound-up spring when I push off and dive in.

To prepare for the dive, I lock my hands and pretend to glue my arm to the sides of my head. It is important my arms and hands stay locked as I lean forward. My fingertips point to where I'll land and if my head becomes unglued from my locked arms, I will belly flop and that can hurt or cause water to go up my nose. Squeezing the back of my ears with my arms will help keep my arms in place.

Before practicing my Seated Dive, I move to deeper water, but always with an adult who can swim.

⚠ WARNING
SHUT the GATE

EYES DOWN!

1.6 m

When I am ready to dive, I take in a Pufferfish Breath, look down and hum as I lean forward and push off the side of the pool with my feet. I straighten my legs out behind me and follow my hands and my body into the water.

As I start to slow down, I unlock my hands and sweep my arms down to my sides. Then I Kick and Flip back to safety.

I CAN DIVE FOR TREASURE !

A fun way to end the class is to go hunting for sunken treasure – diving down to the bottom of the pool to collect sinky toys. Diving for treasure helps me practise a lot of my new swimming skills.

I drop the toys into water that isn't too deep – never throwing the toys, in case I accidently hit someone or break something. Before I Blast Off, I check to see where I am going to dive before I leave the side of the pool or submerged step.

After I Blast Off, I sometimes have to let some of my bubbles out to help me reach the toys. Once I have grabbed a toy, I lower my legs and plant my feet on the floor so I can Blast Off back to the surface with my treasures. To help me spring back faster I blow a huge stream of bubbles on my way back up.

If I am not ready to go to the bottom of the pool, or if I need help, I ask an adult to help me. I can hold their hand and go under with them or they can stand beside the toys and give me a little push to help me reach, until I can do it by myself.

MY ACHIEVEMENTS CHECKLIST

1

I get a little bit better each time I practise my swimming skills.

2

I record my progress using the checklist and a pencil.

3

It reminds me which skills I am really good at and which skills I will need to practise.

4

I know the more I practice the better I will get.

5

When I have practiced and perfected every skill, I know I am ready to move on to Level 3 of Learn to Swim The Australian Way.

	Needs Work	Almost	Perfect
I can do a stride entry			
I can blow bubbles			
I can blow dragon bubbles			
I can zombie float			
I can fly float			
I can dead fly float			
I can frog float			
I can pencil float			
I can blast off			
I can flutter kick			
I can rocket kick			
I can do a soldier float			
I can flip & kick			
I can superman kick			
I can freestyle march			
I can do six kicks switch			
I can caterpillar kick			
I can seahorse balance			
I can do survival backstroke			
I can do a seated dive			
I can dive for treasure			

www.ingramcontent.com/pod-product-compliance
Lightning Source LLC
Chambersburg PA
CBHW040935050426

42334CB00048B/101